AF261041

COVID-19

REAPING WHERE IT DID NOT SOW

A Guide to Understanding the Basics of the Covid-19 Pandemic and Proven Natural Remedies

PRINCE EVANS

Covid-19 Reaping Where It Did Not Sow
A Guide to Understanding the Basics of the Covid-19
Pandemic and Proven Natural Remedies

Paperback ISBN: 978-1-63812-129-9
Hardcover ISBN: 978-1-63812-131-2
Ebook ISBN: 978-1-63812-130-5

Published by Green Sage Agency 09/23/2021

Green Sage Agency
1-888-366-9989
inquiry@greensageagency.com

CONTENTS

INTRODUCTION

I felt a responsibility, sort of a calling, to write an easy and short book that everybody can read to enlighten them about COVID-19 facts I've read in newspapers and scientific studies as understood from a layman's angle. This book is specifically geared toward persuading vaccine skeptics and those who discredit vaccination as the world continues the epic mass vaccination rollout. Nonetheless, it is for a global audience—virtually people of all ages who are able to read. Vaccines of all kinds are made following stringent measures, strictly observing high standards of quality.

COVID-19: Reaping Where It Did Not Sow is basically written to encourage people to take the vaccine, as much as to inform and create awareness for a better understanding of the pandemic with a global view. Its goal is to help readers know the nature of the disease we're dealing with—how to recognize its symptoms, how to limit its rapid spread, why we should contain it, the process of vaccine creation, and what the vaccine and vaccination means. Finally, and most important, it aims to debunk a myriad of *conspiracy theories* suggested by politicians and other skeptics of vaccines to show that vaccines are always safe—that vaccination is neither a ploy to implant tracking microchips into people and experiment on humans nor is it unsafe and lethal This is according to a video by Bill Gates on CBS New website (Gates, 2020).

CHAPTER 1

What Is COVID-19?

COVID-19 is an acronym for a new respiratory viral disease called coronavirus disease of 2019 (SARS-CoV-2), which first originated in Wuhan, China. The disease is believed to be zoonotic, meaning the virus jumped from an animal to humans. It is a highly infectious and potentially fatal disease, especially to the elderly and people with underlying diseases. Specifically, many people with diabetes easily succumb to COVID-19, as well as those with heart conditions or lung conditions. COVID-19 has spread to all parts of the world and is now a global pandemic.

CHAPTER 2

Symptoms of COVID-19

COVID-19 symptoms are wide ranging, from none at all to mild to multiple, causing mild sickness to the dreaded pneumonia. A person can be stable one minute and, in the next, abruptly develops a critical condition. I have heard of close friends waking up symptomless, jovial, and feeling great one morning, but by the end of that day, I get information that they have just dropped dead or are in critical condition at the ICU. According to a study led by researchers from King's College London and reported on Yahoo!'s symptom-tracking COVID-19 study app., there are six types of COVID-19 strains, each distinguished by a particular cluster of symptoms (Sudre, Spector, Ourselin and Steves, 2020). Since the invasion of this viral plague, the symptoms most commonly associated with a COVID-19 infection were fever or chills, cough, sore throat, loss of the senses of taste and smell, loss of appetite, headache, fatigue, congestion or runny nose, nausea or vomiting, diarrhea, muscle and body aches, shortness of breath or difficulty in breathing, and even death. Ironically, these COVID-19 symtoms keep growing not only in number but also in severity! The symptoms can be clustered into six groups. The study found that these group include:

1. Flulike with no fever—headache, loss of smell, muscle pain, cough, sore throat, chest pain
2. Flulike with fever—headache, loss of smell, cough, hoarseness, sore throat, fever, loss of appetite
3. Gastrointestinal—headache, loss of smell, loss of appetite, diarrhea, sore throat, chest pain, no cough
4. Severe level 1, with fatigue—headache, loss of smell, loss of appetite, cough, fever, hoarseness, sore throat, chest pain
5. Severe level 2, with confusion—headache, loss of smell, loss of appetite, cough, fever, hoarseness, sore throat, chest pain, fatigue, muscle pain
6. Severe level 3, with abdominal and respiratory symptoms—headache, loss of smell, loss of appetite, cough, fever, hoarseness, sore throat, chest pain, fatigue, confusion, muscle pain, shortness of breath, diarrhea, abdominal pain

Dr. Claire Steves, the lead researcher, stated that these findings have important implications for care and monitoring of people who are most vulnerable to severe COVID-19.

It has also recently been established that COVID-19 attacks vital organs in the body, depriving them of oxygen and even causing blood clots. "The high levels of d-dimer indicate that the body is trying its darndest to break down the clot," said Dr. Weitz. But "the forces to generate clots are overwhelming the capacity of the body to get rid of them.", a Wall Street article by Daniela Hernandez and Betsy McKay stated that the virus attacks all vital organs in the body leaving it ravaged and deprived of oxygen. Mr. Garvon Russell, a 67-year-old retiree who had been admitted with the COVID-19 Virus at the HMC

Westeinde Hospital in The Hague, said he feels lucky to have survived: "It's nothing to play with." (Hernandez and McKay, 2020)

CHAPTER 3

Containment and Safety Measures

Coronavirus, the virus that causes COVID-19, is a highly infectious disease; thus, it spreads like wildfire. Initially researchers thought it spread through physical contact, such as shaking hands and touching tables, chairs, countertops, and other surfaces contaminated by virus-ridden droplets from our breath. After touching these surfaces, one would rub or touch his or her nose, eyes, or mouth, directly transferring the virus into the body. This is why we are asked not to touch our faces and to frequetnly sanitize or wash our hands with soap and water.

It has recently been found that the virus can also be aerosolized and become airborne. The mists, light enough to float and linger in the air for a substantially long period of time, become airborne transmitters, able to pass the virus to multiple people in a very short time. This finding has been fueled by how rapidly the virus spreads, researchers' observations, and the analysis of recent scientific data. This was also evident through the increase in the number of infections, especially witnessed in the United States in the aftermath of the demonstrations following Fourth of July celebrations and other "superspreader" events, Europe and other parts of the world.

Since this is a new disease, researchers and scientists are learning new trends about it on a daily basis. They analyze data on the fly from the little but vital scientific information coming in whenever research is conducted. For this reason, it is not rare for there to be confusion, conflict of ideas, misinformation, and even reversal of recommendations. This is, in part, because scientists around the world are scrambling, feverishly working overtime, day and night, to learn about the disease, with the goal of developing a vaccine to shield the world from the COVID-19 pandemic. Fortunately, a number of promising vaccine candidates in scientific laboratories around the world have proved promising and will possibly begin to be rolled out to the public by the end of 2020 or in the beginning of the new year.

The main reason for writing this book concern that a lot of us are not informed well enough to understand the disease, its symptoms, and how it spreads. COVID-19 spreads in simple, clear, and normal channels that most of us can easily understand and have the power to stop.

The other reason for this book is to clear the air in a very succinct manner of the doubts many of us have about the safety of vaccines and vaccination. This is because a majority of the world's population do not believe, trust, or understand vaccines because of how they are made or the materials from which they are produced. Reluctance about getting vaccines can also be based on cultural and religious beliefs. My purpose is to assure the world, and mostly vaccine skeptics, that the process of vaccinations has been scientifically proven to be very safe. The making of a vaccine adheres to strict and rigorous efficacy and safety trials and procedures that don't violate anyone's physical well-being or the religious and cultural beliefs of anyone, anywhere.

The Real Reason for Containment Measures

We have seen that the ways in which COVID-19 spreads are common to our basic ways of life, thus making it spread very rapidly from one person to many others in a very short time. Some infected people, in fact, either exhibiting symptoms or asymptomatic have earned the term superspreaders, coined due to the fact these people exhibit herd immunity and can carry the virus for days without feeling the full effects of it, while spreading the virus to huge crowds. This begs the question of not *if* COVID-19 will eventually infect everyone in the world but when it will reach you or me as an individual. We all know it's just a matter of time! Thus, the importance of containment measures to slow the rate of infections by all means possible—modern and sophisticated, rudimentary or archaic. These nonpharmaceutical public health measures now come to play and can neither be overemphasized nor wished away. This is a collective global public responsibility in order for the vaccine to find some of us still breathing.

To keep COVID-19 at bay entails regular scrubbing and washing of hands with enough soap for at least twenty seconds as well as the use of hand sanitizer with at least a 70 percent alcohol base where water and soap is scarce. Putting on a recommended face mask correctly—completely covering the nose and mouth—in any public gathering, whether indoors or outdoors, as well as keeping safe physical social distancing (a minimum of six feet is recommended) and avoiding crowded rooms. Regularly sanitize working surfaces such as tables, chairs, countertops, stands, computer desks, and floors, especially if you have children, elderly people, or individuals with underlying conditions at home. Being careful in following these measures will answer the question of when in the long term. If not well done, the answer could be never!

But what if we do not adhere to the safety measures put in place by and governments?! Is it not strange that, when we make something a habit, that thing becomes second nature to us and, finally, a culture? We do not wear masks because it is our habit and, therefore, our culture not to always have them on. Sound familiar? However, remember that unusual times call for uncommon, often hard decisions and actions. The decision is a resetting of our minds, and the action is the actual effecting of nonpharmaceutical health measures put in place by WHO and governments in our daily lives. COVID-19 has triggered a massive tectonic shift in our ways of life. We just have to reexamine ourselves and repackage how we do our things to effectively deal with it once and for all. After all, what if the making of a vaccine doesn't come to fruition? We've all heard the challenges encompassing the making of it!

A vaccine might seem to be a blessing. And in many ways, it can be. But limited vaccine production infrastructural capacity, general feeble human resource capacity, insensitive and inequitable global channels of distribution, the enormity of physical storage requirements, and the logistics of administration to everyone in the world guarantee that all will be infected before the vaccine gets to them. Even if the vaccine was instantly available in required quantities, the challenge of fairly distributing and safely administering it would be a daunting one. It would take a couple of years for distribution to be 100 percent complete.

This is not just a one-time shot by the way. A vaccine has to be given several times depending on its makeup (for example, one under study requires two injections before it's effective) and how long the vaccine's protection lasts before another is required. For instance, according to US CDC childhood vaccines work very well, but some vaccines, like the flu vaccine, is 40 percent to 60 percent effective depending on the year and the strain of the flu among other things (Centers for Disease Control and Prevention, National Center for Immunization and Respiratory Diseases (NCIRD), 2020).

Even after vaccines are ready and in use, the need for containment measures will not go away overnight. Studies have shown a combination of frequently washing hands with soap and running water thoroughly, maintaining social distancing, correctly wearing a face mask, and avoiding nonessential movements is the bulletproof vest to curbing COVID-19 infection.

CHAPTER 5

The Vaccine-Making Process

Vaccinations are the sure way to treat and even eradicate a target virus, in this case coronavirus, as in the cases of measles and polio. Smallpox and chickenpox are other previously serious viruses that were eradicated by vaccination. We have seen N1H1, an avian virus that caused the 1918 influenza pandemic, wiped off the face of earth. Ebola has been put under control by a vaccine. But HIV/AIDS and the flu are examples of viruses for which a permanent solution or vaccine has been elusive. Vaccines have to be developed and administered to the populous to keep the virus from widely spreading and, particularly, from killing people.

The process of developing a vaccine normally takes years, if not decades! However, this is not going to be the case this time due to the urgency brought about by the nature of COVID-19 pandemic. A vaccine is urgently needed now, and so scientist have raced to come up with one in unbelievably record time. It starts by determining vaccine candidates. There are over 160 COVID-19 vaccine candidates around the world. Some of the leading pharmaceutical companies in the search for COVID-19 vaccine are Oxford University, China's CanSino

Biologic's AdenoVirus, Chinese Sinovac, Novavac, Jonson and Johnson, Moderna and AstraZeneca.

The process involves starting tests for the vaccine on animals such as mice and rabbits first. This is usually followed by lengthy and delicate human trials for a number of years, but normally not exceeding ten. It's then taken through WHO and various government agencies such as FDA for a number of checks and approvals. Mass production and global distribution then takes place. Once a vaccine has been developed and taken by everyone in the world, then we can breathe a sure sigh of relief and go back to our normal way of life as usual! However, production, distribution, and administration of the vaccine is going to take a very long time judging by the sheer numbers of doses needed in order to vaccinate the whole world.

Great efforts by governments and many private multinational organizations have come up with a number of safe and effective vaccines. One of these multinational organizations is the Bill and Melinda Gates Foundation, which is leading the way in terms of funding and the process it takes in COVID-19 virus vaccine development. The process of vaccine development takes years, as it requires strictly adhering to a rigorous step-by-step method that ensures human safety and efficacy of the drug. The task is insurmountable, the will to do it unfathomable, and the funding is only the beginning of it (yet involves mind-boggling numbers). However, Operation Warp Speed (OWS), has anabled the development of a number of vaccines at record time!

Once a vaccine is developed and available for use in case of a pandemic, the sheer numbers involved in the laborious processes of manufacturing, packaging, distribution, and administering the vaccine is mind-boggling to say the least. It would take years for the almost 8 billion global population to be reached. Without blinking an eye, it is safe to say that, by the time the last person is reached, millions more will have died waiting for the vaccine!

So far, despite the safety measures put in place and enforced by governments around the world, the coronavirus pandemic has infected more than 72 million people and counting. More than 1.6 million people have also lost their lives to the deadly virus since it first emerged from China in December 2019, according to a situation report of AFP tally of official sources (AFP, 2020). Something encouraging and that gave hope to those who were at risk and even those infected already was the number of recoveries, which stood at about 2.6 million by March 7, 2020.

There are organizations playing an instrumental role to ensure that we not only get a safe and effective vaccine, but also and equally important that the vaccine be distributed equitably—*globally*! These front-runners include World Health Organization (WHO), the Global Alliance for Vaccines and Immunization (GAVI), and the Bill and Melinda Gates Foundation. This is among thousands of researchers, virologists, and experts in various related fields, all hands on deck for a new COVID-19 vaccine. The WHO plays the critical roles of the collection and dissemination information globally, mobilization of funding, vaccine trial oversight, and facilitation of various vaccine producers in the interest of the whole world. GAVI oversees manufacturing and equitable distribution of the vaccine to the world, including the very vulnerable of the society (GAVI, 2020). The Bill and Melinda Gates Foundation provides expert experience as pertains to vaccine trials and production capacity and is also the largest funder of the global COVID-19 vaccine production and distribution once it's ready for use.

CHAPTER 6

Patient Zero around the World

The severe acute respiratory syndrome (SARS-CoV-2), coronavirus of 2019 (COVID-19) disease, like many other global plagues felt like aliens furiously attacking humans to reclaim the world for their selfish ends. A virus characteristically unique from other viruses before, mainly by the nature of its symptoms and rapid spread of infections, COVID-19 fueled this frantic search for patient zero whenever it was suspected that the virus had percolated into any city or country. But more specifically, who was really "patient zero" for the outbreak?

Also known as an index case, patient zero is a common terminology used to describe the first human to be infected by a viral or a bacterial disease in an outbreak. In the case of COVID-19 pandemic, the *Wall Street Journal* identified a fifty-seven-year-old woman by the name Wei Guixian, a seller of shrimp at the Huanan Seafood Market on December 10, when she developed the cold (Fan, Page and Khan, 2020). Patient zero proved important in various ways. With any communicable disease, finding patient zero proves important in various ways. For one, he or she is the key pertaining to the origin of the outbreak. Contact tracing originating from this patient could carry on down to the last man in the chain. In the case of Wuhan, finding patient zero was of paramount importance not only to know how the virus was born but also to curb the spread of the virus through the same means. Every time there was a single positive diagnosis, a swift chase for contacts was initiated. This proved extremely difficult, and late in the game, the virus had gotten out of hand and crossed the borders.

In some instances, the contacts would be really difficult to find, and even if found, they proved stubborn. Technology was developed around this activity based on the smartphone as a tracking device. There was also technology developed for self-check that allowed people to answer a series of question through an application of a web page, such as Facebook. Many of the people who found out they could have been infected shied away from declaring their status for fear of victimization and stigmatization by family, friends, and neighbors.

In Kenya, patient zero was a woman by the name Brenda Cherotich. According to NikkoTunui of The Standard News Paper, this first case of COVID-19 was reported and known to the public on March 13, 2020, long after the first case in Wuhan, China (Tanui, 2020). Brenda a twenty-seven-year-old woman had traveled from the United States via London, United Kingdom, arriving in Kenya on March 5, 2020. At first on her arrival in Kenya, she wasn't aware that she was sick, and only later did she begin feeling unwell. By this time, she had been up and about visiting family and friend in the city of Nairobi. She had even attended a party at a house in Ongata Rongai, on the outskirts of Nairobi. One of those she had been with was a guy by the name Brian Orinda, who was established as the third patient. Brenda was first thought to be a student travelling back to Kenya to visit her family. She latter clarified that she was not a student but former Kericho Model and had travelled to Ohio to represent her family at her elder brother Patrick Ngetich's graduation ceremony.

In some quarters, it was viewed as an attack! Point in case, in the United States, the search for patient zero turned into a conspiracy-theory fiasco, with a great number of malicious people going after the blood of an individual believed to be patient zero, accusing her of bringing the virus to the United States as a biological weapon. However, it is not very well known when exactly the virus hit the United States, since the discovery of pateint 0 and government response was way off the mark by weeks after the invasion. According to an article in *Medpage Today* based on a forensic pathologist's investigation, Santa Clara, California, public health officials discovered that SARS-CoV-2, the virus that causes COVID-19, was responsible for the death of Patricia Down, an apparently asymptomatic fifty-seven-year-old woman who worked in Silicon Valley and who died on February 6, 2020, of cardiac tamponade from a ruptured heart (Melinek, 2020). Since then, about nine deaths that had not been classified as COVID-19 deaths have been reclassified as COVID-19 deaths. So, in the United States, the first death to be cited as a COVID-19 death was that of the Santa Clara woman known as Patricia Down. However, Down's autopsy report, according to Dr. Judy Melinek, a forensic pathologist and Investigator demonstrates that this patient zero assumption is almost certainly wrong and many weeks off the mark! Down's death from COVID-19 is one of the very few rare cases of very healthy normal people with no history of medical preconditions of any kind succumbing to the illness.

The medic goes on to say that, for a normal adult, the weight of the heart is about 290 grams. Down's heart was right on the mark. Her heart was also of normal shape. Nonetheless, the autopsy showed that the muscle tissues had been badly damaged—enough that the left ventricular wall had torn open. A heart will typically suffer this kind of severe damage in the setting of high blood pressure and high cholesterol, in patients who have had prior myocardial infarction.

These aftereffects, in some instances, lasted for weeks or months on ends. In general, full recovery wasn't guaranteed, and that was the beginning of everything going south. Symptoms varied from person to person, with some having mild to no symptoms at all, while others experienced severe symptoms. If there is any lesson to learn, we could draw from the incredible speed at which this virus spread that humans are very highly interconnected, interrelated, and interdependent on each other. We live as one. There is no sole actor in all our spheres of life. And in actuality, we live *for* one another.

Despite a stream of strange scientifically unconfirmed guesses, such as that the virus doesn't infect African people or that it kills older people more than younger people, COVID-19 continued to spread quickly into the African community, and a few older people luckily survived. On the other hand, most younger people who were mistakenly thought to have a strong immune system were also felled by the pandemic. It was a global thing.

Every part of the world—be it Asia, Europe, North America, South America, Africa, or Australia—has been hit, with all the races in the world being infected and devastatingly affected indiscriminately. Believe me, if Antarctica was a habitable continent, it wouldn't have been spared from the virus.

There is a notable difference that can be found in many countries of Africa, where the virus has fared differently than it has in the more developed parts of the world. Although disadvantaged economically, many African countries were better of in terms of the spread of the virus. Key facts have played a crucial role in the lowering of the spread of the pandemic. First is the minimal and poorly constructed infrastructural development, which in turn discourages and cuts down on the level of movement of people. As we all know, any pandemic is fueled by movement. Due to the minimum levels of movement of people, the virus has lacked the fuel to swiftly grip the population and take root in Africa. So, the peak, for example in Kenya, is still a long way to come, and when and where it peaked won't likely be known for a very long time.

The other fact is that very few people in Africa own motorized means of movement. The daily mode of movement is walking, even with lack of sidewalks on the streets. In some communities, people walk for tens of miles to fetch basic commodities like water and food. A few use bicycles. Many use public transportation and sometimes motorbikes. Even then, travel isn't relatively far in terms of distances. Pandemically speaking, this is a huge advantage! Economically speaking, it's a huge disadvantage! Even manual bicycles are owned by very few people, and even those who have them don't go very far. In other words, most everyday activities in these villages are localized, and so there's rarely an exchange between distant villages. Where there is, the exchange is very light. Life in African villages is very slow in comparison to life in Western countries.

Unlike in Asia and Europe, there are no high-speed trains in Africa, a mode of transportation used to move people massively, incredibly at lightning speed. The webs and interconnection of infrastructure are not only massive but also smooth and very impressive. The movements are really effortless. But then, apart from the economical expense, the pandemic fueled by the micro corona virus is the recent highest unseen expense, even though it's brought the whole world to a standstill.

Moreover, there is the fastest mode of communication, and that is airplanes. In a normal day in normal times, in a given minute in the United States, there are thousands of airplanes in the air moving thousands of people every day. Cutting that to almost zero abruptly was a shock to humanity, though as most environmentalists observed, it was a drastic improvement for the quality of precious air and the clarity of the amazing blue skies—a boost to efforts to slow global warming and increase environmental cleanliness.

However, one group of people the virus doesn't beat up as hard is women. If there is anything sexist about this disease, then this virus would earn the label "against men"! For men, God forbid you get the virus. It's harder for men not only to heal from COVID-19 but also to survive it. It's generally estimated that 5 percent of all the people infected with COVID-19, unfortunately, pass on.

At the forefront are the generals are the medical personnel, such as the nurses, doctors, cleaning staff, and other hospital support staff. The majority of these fallen soldiers are educated, hardworking, caring, loving men who have left their families devastated.

What mattered was that it was a global pandemic and that it needed to be arrested as quickly as possible. The fight against the pandemic that was threatening the lives of the whole world was on a few months after its first diagnosis; the world was undeterred in its pursuit to furiously crush it—at least serious governments were. At this point, thousands were being infected daily, thousands more were losing their lives, and those who miraculously recovered came out of weaker and sometimes seriously disabled by the intrusive nature of ventilators and other hospital equipment used on them. Specialists observed that contracting the virus was the end for the unlucky ones with severe preexisting conditions, especially diabetes and high blood pressure, and those of old age.

Patient zero was the initial originator of COVID-19 pandemic in the case of Wuhan, China. The very first, most sought individual by the Chinese authorities was eventually reported in December 2019. Many people had mixed feelings for this person in whom the virus had originated—anger, confusion, remorse, sadness, rage, and hate! These feelings came in spite of the fact that, despite being the initial virus carrier, she had no purposeful intention to get millions of people globally sick! It is believed that the virus jumped from a bat to humans (that it's zoonotic).

However, as the virus continued infecting and spreading, "patient zero" wore many cultural and racial faces across the globe. In every country, it was believed that the first person to acquire the virus had flown the virus in from either Asia (China) or Europe. Being the first patient came with its fair share of problems, such as blame and shame that were uncalled for. In the United States, it was a woman who got the virus in Wuhan first. For her, she was also suspected, presumed to be a spy and a criminal suspect. In Wuhan, patient zero was maliciously thought to have gotten the virus from making a meal of a bat that was infected with the virus. That was the theory of how the virus initially began that went around the world like wildfire.

CHAPTER 7

Hospitals' Response to COVID-19

To say the least, there wasn't a hospital system in the world that could have handled the shock that COVID-19 brought to society! In a matter of days of the discovery and quarantine of a symptomatic patient zero in a country, there would be an influx of COVID-19 patients in the hospitals. Scientists discovered that a person who has just contacted SARS-CoV-2 cannot test positive for the virus right away; it can, instead, take up to five days before an infection can be discovered by testing. A person would be symptomatic eleven days later and onward. However, before this time, the asymptomatic person would be going about daily activities as usual, without anyone around him or her noticing he or she was sick. All the while, the person would be infecting everyone around him or hin. One person could infect hundreds of people depending on the person's activities, whether a mother of school-going children, a shopper, a manager who uses public transportation to get to work daily, a trader at a market, and so on!

By the end of the incubation period, the whole community would be sick without anyone of them noticing. The creepy damage of this disease is that this was a serious and troubling phenomenon around Asia, Europe, and North America in the first few months of the disease, silently destroying society from within out. Symptoms, for those who were brought in, ranged from severe to serious to mild. Nevertheless, the extent of care afforded the patients and the manner in which hospitals handled all cases was similar, for the danger and consequences of not doing so was of equal measure.

Hospitals were overwhelmed in every respect. Case in point was the New York City (NYC) hospital system, which saw a surge in patients within weeks. Hospital rooms were limited, resulting in an overflow in the general wards and emergency rooms. In most instances, COVID-19 patients would be lined up in hospital hallways or left in the ER, waiting for an open intensive care unit (ICU) bed to open up. ICU overflow resulted in the creation of two emergency makeshift hospitals in New York's Central Park and Javits Convention Center (CNBC New, 2020).

Following this surprising expansion, there also came a shortage of all sorts of medics, including doctors, lab technicians, pharmacists, therapists, and nurses who took care of the patients. These medics were highly threatened by the situation, largely due to a shortage of personal protective equipment (PPE). Three types of vital medical supplies were in high demand and yet very scarce—PPE, ventilators, and testing kits. In the United States, the shortages of ventilators led to state governors pleading with the federal government to intervene. The central government generally lacked coherent messaging and coordination to curb the spread of the pandemic from Washington, DC. This resulted in soaring infection rates and deaths in the United States.

In South Africa, about three months into the scourge, things had unraveled and literally gone south, yet the peak of the infection was nowhere in sight. The first case was confirmed by the Ministry of Health on March 5, 2020, with the first known case being a male South African citizen who had just arrived from Italy. According to *Wikipedia*, the first death to have occurred from COVID-19 pandemic was reported on March 27, 2020 (LSGH, 2020). Just like other countries, South Africa grappled with city- and country-wide lockdowns, shortage of PPE and hospital ICU beds, shortage of all kinds of medical personnel, and mismanagement of messaging of control measures to the public.

These measures did not bear good fruits, as the spread spiraled across the country with the first death of the virus being reported on March 27, 2020. South Africa became the country in Africa with the highest number of COVID-19 pandemic infections, securing position five among countries with highest numbers of infections globally—behind the United States, Brazil, Russia, and India—albeit with relatively low death rates. Just like any other country in the world, South Africa had to strike a balance between the people's livelihood (the economy) and the lockdowns (safety and security of the people) to curb the spread of the pandemic. In April and May 2020, South Africa imposed a strict lockdown that actually slowed down the rate of infections dramatically. However, the lockdown wreaked havoc, causing much economic damage and forcing the government to gradually reopen in June.

At one point, the South African government caved in to complaints of mismanagement of hospital resources, including allegations of widespread corruption during its response to the pandemic as reported by BBC News (Dartnell, 2020). In one situation, it was reported that, to manage the huge numbers of COVID-19 patients, tents became a solution for the high influx of patients. The tents where not set up observing the standards for taking care of sick people. In one such case, a doctor turned whistleblower at Sebokeng Hospital lamented, "It was freezing in that tent. As soon as night falls, it's horrible, you can see the patients declining. Hypothermia is one of the major causes of death here. Especially in that tent." The doctor went to say that, in one forty-eight-hour-period, fourteen people had reportedly died in the tents but not all of them due to hypothermia. The doctor continued to describe the "horrific" scenes in the marquee-sized tent set up in the car parking lot and used by the hospital as a makeshift triage and waiting room. This was over the course of cold and hectic weeks in July, with elderly patients collapsing after being left for two days or more without sanitation, food, or proper heating. Sick people were forced to crowd around three small old electric heaters that frequently broke. There was also an acute shortage of drugs and ventilator equipment. It was reported that there was used PPE lying all over the place, waiting to infect more people, and actually a number of medical staff had been infected by the virus due to the deplorable conditions.

Just like many other countries in the world and especially African countries, another pandemic was wiping out people in equal measure to the COVID-19 pandemic. This was the corruption that has always been a deadly vice in governments. This time, though it was worsened and its effects made more pronounced by the pandemic. In one instance in South Africa, Jeanette Mlombo, whose son, Martin, had died at the Sebokeng Hospital at the age of thirty said that it was corruption and carelessness that had led to her son's death. She said, "It was freezing. He was shivering, starving. I slept the whole night here at the tent without any blanket. I am going to die. Nobody's taking care of me." Ms. Mlombo recalled her conversation with her son. In a letter addressed to all of the ruling party of the Africa National Congress (ANC) members, President of South African Cyril Ramaphosa appeared to take responsibility when he delivered a withering message regarding a controversy surrounding the awarding of contracts to help the country deal with the COVID-19 pandemic to influential people in the government.

In India, the government unveiled a thousand-bed capacity makeshift hospital in Mumbai on April 2020 in preparation for the surge of COVID-19 pandemic patients in the country. The makeshift Wuhan-style hospital was built by Mumbai Metropolitan Region Development Authority (MMRDA) at Bandra-Kurla Complex in the commercial capital of India as a quarantine and an isolation facility for COVID-19 patients. Unlike the South African temporary hospitals, the Mumbai facility featured a pathological laboratory, oxygen facilities, and cabins for doctors and nurses, as well as other facilities. India did not stop there; it went ahead and unveiled another mega makeshift hospital in New Delhi to accommodate COVID-19 patients—this one with a capacity of ten thousand. The sprawling tent, measuring 1,700 feet by 700 feet, is petitioned into two hundred sections that can fit fifty beds each. It's complete with air coolers, a staff of over a thousand health care professionals, oxygenation units, and two large toilet complexes on either side of the mega tent. The hospital started operation in early July.

The first case of the COVID-19 pandemic in India, which has the largest number of COVID-19 victims in Asia, was reported on January 30, 2020, and is believed to have originated from China. India has the third highest number of infections in the world after the United States and Brazil, with over a million confirmed cases by July 17, 2020.

CHAPTER 8

Treatment of COVID-19

There are no cures for COVID-19. It being a brand-new disease, there are no medications for it of any kind anywhere in the world. As we continue dealing with this pandemic, people talked about using remedies and medication meant for other diseases, such as antiretrovirals meant for AIDS and hydroxychloroquine meant for malaria. However, as warned by many doctors and scientists, these medications could have adverse side effects, causing bodily chemical and physical injury. The least such medications could do was to have no form of negative bodily effects at all, which is a better outcome considering the two options.

However, how do you know that the medication is not working? If one is still hurting with symptoms of COVID-19 after taking a medicine that does not work, he or she may be waiting to be better when, in truth, he or she is dying! This is why medicine developments undergo rigorous scientific studies and trials.

Before medications are introduced to the public for use, their developers have to follow scientifically proven tests, studies, and procedures for safety and efficacy. Testing of a vaccine or drug for safety begins by testing it on animals such as mice. This process ensures the medication is safe (if it doesn't kill the mice). Safety tests ensure that treatments or vaccinations do not have adverse side effects that can lead to the users' long-term or permanent disabilities. Efficacy procedures ensure the medication cures what it is supposed to treat and to what percentage fitness or effectiveness. For example, if a vaccine clears 100 percent of the virus, then it is very good. A 50 percent effective treatment of the targeted disease leaves the sick still hurting and symptomatic. This means that the vaccine may be administered in several doses or a different approach or vaccine should be used.

The other form of treatment considered was the use of antibodies. Antibodies are the protein the body makes to fight off infections. According to CNN, scientsts have harnessed this natural protection for treatment since the Victorian era (Christensen, 2020). This process has been applied very successfully to bacterial infections and some viral infections. However, it's not very effective when applied to viruses. Antibodies also enable the basic standard for discovering whether people have been infected or not. If antibodies are detected in blood samples, then the person is either sick or was once infected but has been cured of the virus. The absence of antibodies simply means that no infection has occurred yet. With antibodies-based treatment, you have to contract the virus first and survive it. The antibodies you develop provide some form of immunity to the body for some limited time frame. Once antibodies are detected, convalescent plasma is drawn to extract antibodies that are then used for treatment of other people after processing.

This is the use of the body's own immune mechanism, working to cure itself after developing antibodies. However, like any other process, use of antibodies to check the status of sickness may not work or can be flawed. There is always a chance of a false negative or a false positive.

On top of that, there is always fraudulent effort by unscrupulous actors out to make a quick buck, taking advantage of the fear, anxiety, and confusion in the health industry by intentionally manufacturing faulty antibody testing kits. They use the fear of the pandemic as an opportunity to take advantage of the populous by swindling them. COVID-19 has not been an exception with these fraudsters. They have been working day and night to perfect their trickery, making enormous quick kills. Faulty test kits will result in a false negative or a false positive outcome!

A false negative result means that the tested person is sick, but the test shows otherwise. This can be really serious, since the person could still be either asymptomatic, the testing kit could be faulty, or the testing procedures could be flawed. Although the asymptomatic person is usually energetic and going about business as usual, he or she is a superspreader of the COVID-19 virus. And by the time such a person starts exhibiting symptoms, he or she would have spread the virus to thousands of people, starting from loved ones and friends. From here, the spread is exponential, reaching the whole community, as those family and friends go about their daily duties oblivious of their health status. Asymptomatic people do not see the need to take any precaution, since they feel healthy. That could mean that such a person wouldn't take any remedy or take required preventative measures, and therefore, he or she would continue infecting others until showing the symptoms and being quarantined, tested, and isolated.

On the other hand, asymptomatic COVID-19 patients who've undergone treatment can be superspreaders as well. When quarantined and tested positive, they still may have no COVID-19 symptoms at all, though they may be infected and actively spreading. Due to viral mutation, the virus manifests in different people differently by varied symptoms. Some may be seriously sick with all kinds of symptoms, while others may experience mild symptoms with no pain at all.

Then there is the case of a false positive test result. This is when the results show the person is sick when the person is actually as fit as a fiddle. If all resources are available and proper procedures are followed, this is the person who could end up on a stretcher in an ambulance and on a hospital bed in an isolation center full of COVID-19 patients unnecessarily. It is a scary situation to contemplate, as this person could be wrongfully quarantined or even isolated together with sick people. In this environment, one is automatically at high risk of contracting the infection!

At the same time, there were reports from a few African countries where ordinary people, medicine men, and even political leaders and government officials encouraged citizens to use different sorts of concoctions for cure. According to BBC News Online, one prominent example is when the Madagascar's president, Andry Rajoelina, around May 5, 2020, promoted the use of herbal concoctions called herbal tonic for treatment of COVID-19 patients (BBC, 2020). This action was met by a condemnation against the use of the herbal tonic by WHO and African Union (AU). The two international organizations specifically condemned the use of the herbs, firmly stating that any substance used as a cure for COVID-19 must undergo scientific safety and efficacy screening before use. However, with the herbal tonic, this was not done to the standards used to test vaccines and other medicine.

A test for chemical toxicity was carried out in Germany, which found out that, although the herbal concoction was not poisonous, it had no medicinal effects or value in the treatment of COVID-19 on patients. Despite this outcome, the president of Madagascar continued to popularize the herbal tonic. He went as far as sending free supplies to a number of African countries, which included South Africa, Tanzania,

Democratic Republic of Congo, Guinea Bissau, Liberia, Central Africa Republic, and Equatorial Guinea.

There is also the case of an herbal remedy in Kenya that hasn't made rounds in the media yet it is a licensed product. Because this is being undertaken by the Kenya Medical Research Institute (KEMRI), a government parastatal through the appropriate channels, the biggest hindrance to mass production has been funding. The herb, known as Zedupex, is a traditional medicine normally known in Kenya to remedy genital herpes. There is a lot of promise and hope around this traditional remedy. WHO was prompted to announce that it had called for a meeting of seventy traditional herbal medicine experts across Africa to deliberate on the role of traditional medicine in response to the COVID-19 pandemic. According to the Kenyan *Daily Nation*, the organization unanimously resolved that clinical trials must be conducted on all medicines in the region, without exception (Nation Online, 2020).

On about June 16, 2020, a medication that was proved to reduce death in severely infected COVID-19 patients was discovered. Early studies showed that the steroid dexamethasone reduced death in over a third of patients with severe COVID-19. This was very surprising but very good news for the world. Given enough of this steroid, the rate of deaths caused by the relentless COVID-19 pandemic would drastically be reduced, and the world would soon go back to normalcy very quickly. This medication has proved to be just a remedy for covid-19 since it just slows down the rate of infection and the pain inflicted by the virus but does not totally clear it. This is typical of viruses! With the discovary of vaccines, it is going to play a greater role in slowing down the virus, the pain and consiquently deaths as we wait for the distribution of vaccines across the world.

CHAPTER 9

The Community Fear of COVID-19

Talking about real, well-founded fear in relation to COVD-19 is an understatement. Fear was everywhere; in every aspect of life; and for every person, rich or poor, strong or weak, fat or thin, tall or short, all over the world. There was fear of falling sick with other illnesses and ending up in hospital, only to come in contact with COVID-19. There was fear of flying, which meant you would be confined in an airplane for lengthy periods of time in close proximity with people who you knew nothing about—neither their health condition nor where they came from. Flying also meant that one would end up quarantined in the country of destination, for fourteen days in a number of countries, before being released to proceed within his or her touchdown country. There was fear that, in the case one ended up in quarantine, he or she would be released only after being tested and confirmed negative and after paying for accommodation for the fourteen days. There was fear of losing the freedom of going shopping without contracting the virus. There was fear of losing jobs, which was rampant. Some company executives took advantage of the opportunity to lay people off, even if the claims they made about reasons for laying them off was unfounded. There was fear of losing business due to fewer customers or, in some cases, no customer at all.

This was what going shopping meant—putting on a mask and enduring the heat inside the car or walking the streets and enduring the sweat! Maintaining social distancing was easy to say but tough to do. Unconsciously, people would find themselves in very close proximity to each other, as being close to others had always been the norm. Coughing or sneezing in an elbow sounded easy; however, combined with all other measures, it felt like an insurmountable mountain to scale! There was fear surrounding every minor, regular activity of daily living—tasks as simple as hand washing or hand sanitizing that people had previously taken for granted!

All this fear led to a number of leaders quipping that, since we lived in abnormal times brought about by the coronavirus, we should act abnormally. This meant that we must keep strict social distance, mask our faces, stay at home, sanitize ourselves, and constantly wash our hands with soap and clean running water. If we didn't act abnormally paranoid about these actions, the virus would force us into submission! People's fears were founded in the fact that this virus was not only highly contagious but also fatal and permanently injurious as seen in many cases. In terms of numbers, by May 6, 2020, there were 1,588,773 people infected and 247,503 people confirmed dead globally. The rate of infections was worryingly very high (WHO, 2020).

Yet by this time, people had gotten tired of being confined in their homes already, after over a month of very strict containment measures from governments. It was very exhausting; it was financially draining and psychologically devastating. Governments world over had to strike a balance between lives and livelihoods, which was really difficult for many countries, especially developing economies where most people live from hand to mouth and have to fetch daily bread on a daily basis. Whenever the government eased the restrictions, people would let loose and stop observing the safety measures put in place. This would fuel the fire of the spread of infections, and in a matter of two weeks, there would be another spike and deaths. This would worry the government, which would, therefore, order another lockdown or cessation of movement.

However, for the most part, the change was positive, inevitable, and here to stay for the long haul—probably for eternity. After six months into the virus, scientists and other experts and even the general public gave in to the fact that life the way we knew it had come to an end. A new dawn had unexpectedly arrived. The workplace routine as we knew it was flipped up to its belly, with most companies moving to virtual, or rather remote, work or meetings.

CHAPTER 10

The Inevitable Changes to Our Lives

Going forward, we would still need to maintain social distancing in the short term to medium term to control the exponential spread of coronavirus. Workplaces using hot desk toping would need to reconsider that workplace arrangement and maybe go back to a more traditional office arrangement, where one man or woman uses a traditional one door, brick-and-mortar office. Huge office spaces occupied by employees in the hundreds at a time would be hotbeds for virus exchange. The era of cubicles with countless employees' heads popping above the wooden or plastic petitions seemed to become a thing of the past, as we smelled change in the air, blown in by the COVID-19 pandemic.

Along with these pricey physical structural changes, social and cultural changes that may be more permanent will follow suit. These are the more enduring kinds of changes, becoming the norm or the culture. Not forgetting that culture, once entrenched, niether disappoints nor dies out! For example, the telemarketing industry, the call centers, and the factory floors will face a huge transformative change. This has already partly come, in the form of work schedules of various forms, including working in shifts around the clock or working from home. This may eventually and permanently lead to a shift in expectations and workplace culture, where employers are valued on how they perform in terms of manner of communication, punctuality, and timely deliverables and not their physical punctuality to the office and how late they leave office, how long they sit behind their desks, or even whether or how long they go to lunch. The norm of getting up early, arriving at work at 8:00 a.m.; and staying until 5:00 p.m. may disappear for some industries altogether.

The effects of these changes will translate to a drastic reduction in the movements of people, translating to less public transportation as well as private cars on city streets but more people walking. Well, you guessed right; this now leads us into economic downsizing. Think about it for a minute. There will be few people buying cars. As a result, people will revert to bicycling; use of electronic scooters, roller boards, and roller skates; and many other such modes of transportation.

Transportation or travelling as we know it has essentially changed, may it be for the good of the environment or for the worst of humanity! This will affect both short-distance and long-distance travel. Transport by rail, road or airplane went down by almost 20 percent or even more in terms of capacity. Electric scooters, previously banned in the United Kingdom, may be legalized again. Some cities have started encouraging people to either walk or cycle, for example cities in the United Kingdom or the United States. For many African countries, already basically and largely walking economies, there may not be a big change. In fact, most of the previously mentioned countries have started restricting how their citizens move around their cities. They are doing this by widening streets and creating extra lanes for bikes, scooters, and Rollerblades, transforming how people move.

Life is what happens around you when you least expect it; minute by minute, we experience these changes that we intend to live with for ages. Sometimes the change may be a force of nature, as in the earth rotating west to east on its axis. Even those powerful global leaders who are event influencers have to adapt to the forces of nature and life as it is now and as probably will be in the long run. The COVID-19 pandemic is synonymous with the rotation of the earth, the force of nature.

Positive social, economic, and environmental changes have been brought about by the COVID-19 pandemic. These changes will definitely and positively be felt on a grand scale as we try to force ourselves back to normalcy. Economically, real estate may be headed to a drastically reduced value as workers hunker down in their houses to avoid infections. Some buildings may degrade and end up crumbling and wasteful, due to underutilization or not being utilized at all. Leasing office space may be a thing of the past. Workers may no longer need to remain within commuting distance of the office but, rather, may choose to live wherever is most convenient for them or just anywhere they like. Due to downsizing, more people will move to the suburbs, countryside, or rural areas for those with farms there. This will be the reversal of the industrial revolution era, where people moved to cities in search of employment.

Since there are no factories in the rural areas, people would default to farming and small-scale businesses. Due to this, a number of factories would close down, leading to a reduction of greenhouse gases. We could be headed to those days of tranquility in the air, with less or even no traffic, calmer and safer roads, clean fresh air, fresh clean water, fewer sewerage plants to deal with in the cities, and a quieter environment. Freely moving wild and domestic animals on city streets would be a common thing. And this pandemic, in that sense, has provided an opportunity to reconsider the green economy, providing us a view to how a greener earth might feel or what it might look like otherwise disaster abides in the not-too-distant future if we maintain the status quo such as global temperature rising, sea level rising resulting to disastrous weather events. Included in the environmental changes that have happened for the few months since the pandemic started, data from satellites have shown a 30 to 40 percent reduction in nitrogen dioxide gas, a key component in global warming, and lessening of sooty particles in the air, which, like nitrogen dioxide, also causes respiratory diseases. This has probably already saved the lives of tens or even thousands of people.

According to BBC Online, Scientists have also estimated that the global economic slowdown brought about by coronavirus pandemic is estimated to reduce global carbon dioxide by 8 percent (Dartnell, 2020). If this reduction remains the same for a decade or more, it would result in reduction of global warming to the level of preindustrial temperatures as desired and stipulated in the Paris Agreement. This would be an achievement toward a global warming fix, although it doesn't feel and look like the long-term effects on the environment of global warming poses an immediate greater threat than the short-term emergency of the COVID-19 pandemic. We can also say that lack of action on global warming is a lack of commitment to our future generations and a sign that we don't care whether they survive or die.

We've long seen the great power of national governments working to pressure humanity in multiple ways. For the pandemic, the task was relatively straightforward—getting the general public to recognize that there is a clear and present danger and, thus, to accept the intervention necessary to keep themselves and their loved ones, as well as their wider community, safe. However, the problem with climate change is that it is a more gradual, less visible or less felt process, with less direct link to deaths in developed countries.

CHAPTER 11

Political Influence

The pandemic brought disruptions in all spheres of life. It wasn't just a health issue, it also turned out to be a political issue at various points as well! In fact, in the early stages of COVID-19, some leaders compared its effects and damage to be less disruptive than previous viral infections such as the 1918 influenza epidemic, the H1N1 flu of 2009, Ebola, and others. Politically, there were intrigues all over the world, although it was a war to be won on its own effort and merit politically. No one could guess that there were incredibly big political wars playing in the undercurrent of the unrelenting virus, for it had overtaken all the news headlines in all leading global media houses.

In the United States, election campaigns were warming up! President Donald Trump was fighting for reelection in his naturally unwavering, confusing, and rhetorical political way. He was running against Joe Biden, a political powerhouse in the United States and former vice president to former President Barack Obama. With Trump came unbelievable comics, theatrics, satire, and minimization or inflation of daily media briefings. The lack of seriousness was akin to neglect of duty brought about by a combination of ignorance and lack of political exposure or experience, not to mention a carefree attitude! Trump is a politician whose very nature is self-defeating, in terms of his self-infliction of damage to his reputation as a leader—anyhow, anywhere, and any time he speaks. He had just undergone an intense impeachment process and now the coronavirus pandemic hit; it was like the adage, "Out of the frying pan into the fire!" According to BBC News Online, a vivid example of this is when he addressed the whole world, suggesting that people could treat themselves with hydroxychloroquine or injest bleach—that it knocked the virus out of the system in minutes (BBC.COM News, 2020). This was unbelievable coming from the leader of the free world!

A few weeks later, he was at it again, suggesting that disinfectants such as Lysol and Clorox clear the virus when injected into the body. At the same briefing, he insinuated that the sun could clear the virus, like a joke, if scientists could find a way of beaming it into the body (BBC.COM News, 2020).

The killing of George Floyd on May 25, 2020, by a police officer got tens of thousands of protesters on the streets of major cities across the United States of America. The protests became a norm—peaceful by the day and violent, destructive, and lawless by the night. They also became megaspreader events, since most protesters didn't observe safety measures as simple as mask wearing. Floyd was killed by a white police officer, Derek Chauvin, who put his knee on Floyd's neck for almost nine minutes while Floyd pleaded for his life shouting "I can't breathe." After the video of the incident came out, all four officers were dismissed and charged in court with various offenses, including third-degree murder for Derek Chauvin.

The presumptive democratic presidential nominee and contender against Trump for the presidency and a veteran of politics was Joe Biden, after a very competitive democratic primary. Trump was glaring at losing the White House after almost daily hard-to-believe missteps coming from a US president. Biden condemned the incident, and in the coming weeks, he would unveil Kamala Harris as his vice-presidential choice for the elections. Political battlefields reverted virtually, fearfully due to the deadly COVID-19 pandemic. The Democratic National Convention, popularly known as the DNC, took place virtually, followed by the Republican National Convention (RNC) the following week.

In Kenya, unlike in the United States, there were no elections on the way. But the politics of reviewing the constitution, known as BBI, were at play. The politics of constitution mending and referendum was in the air, and it felt just like a general election was around the corner. The Building Bridges Initiative (BBI) frenzy had been cut short by social distancing measures put in place and enforced by the government. The atmosphere was charged with politics, albeit underground, as privileged political figure in similitude to The Animal Farm, trotted from county to county despite the cessation of movements around the country. A political truce had just been struck between de facto opposition leader Raila Odinga, who had just been appointed the special envoy of Infrastructure Development in Africa, and the incumbent President Uhuru Kenyatta— famously referred to as the handshake. The handshake resulted in the public perception that president Kenyatta appeared to be throwing his deputy president, Dr. William Ruto, under the bus, leading to an outcry among his ardent followers, the Tanga Tanga! The Kieleweke, as opposed to the William Ruto wing of Tanga Tanga political formation, was in support of the Uhuru government. Accusations and counteraccusations against each other were made in the political arena, each defending his position—and all of it available for public consumption. The division of revenue among the counties in the senate was such an argument that it took a very long time for the parties to come to an agreement.

In Europe, Brexit was hot off the political cooking oven, causing economic confusion and meltdown. The United Kingdom worried about its currency, travelers were confused that they would be locked in airports due to lack of travel documents, and all worried that prices of basic services and goods would go through the roof. British Prime Minister Boris Johnson was slow to respond and give direction to the nation. Even as late as March, when the virus was well reported in many countries around the world, London staged an England-Wales rugby match on March 7, 2020, attended by 81,000 fans, together with the prime minister himself as the cheerleader. On March 11, 52,000 mega-spreader events of soccer fans watched Liverpool play Atletico Madrid. For the Cheltenham Festival, one of the country's poshest steeplechase festivals, which ended on March 13, 252,000 punters went to celebrate.

When Johnson did respond, it was a false start, by adopting a strategy of COVID-19 isolation and heard immunity, rather than taking the approach of testing. Boris Johnson's ignorance and inability to grasp the seriousness of the pandemic in February was at its highest when he intentionally chose not to attend meetings of the emergency ministerial group COBRA. The attitude of Mr. Johnson and his unwillingness to get appropriate advice and get ahead of the game has haunted the United Kingdom's efforts to combat this deadly virus ever since.

This slow start has helped explain why the pandemic is rampant in nursing homes for the elderly, why medics and caregivers are scrambling for PPE and there is never enough, and why Britian is way behind other European nations that are mapping the virus through testing and tracking through contact tracing. While Britons were getting together to amuse themselves at mega-spreader events, Europe was shutting down. Borders were closing, and public gatherings were being banned. Italy went into a full lockdown on March 9, 2020;

Denmark, on March 11; Spain, on March 14; and France, on March 15. This wasn't followed by the British until March 23, 2020!

In Brazil, President Jair Bolsonaro was brazened with his response to reporters when asked if he cared that the country was going to be another ground zero behind China due to his ignorance. Bolsonaro minimized the situation and the severity of COVID-19 as the number of cases and deaths ticked upward unabated. By around April 24, 2020, it was estimated that cases of infections in Brazil had reached a million. With a cavalier attitude like this, it was unbelievable that the number of infections were accurate as well, let alone the number of deaths! He contradicted his government health appointees by scoffing at measures put in place, such as social distancing, washing of hands, and putting on masks, retorting publicly, "We will all die one day." He doubled it down by calling on all citizens to go back to work, in effect going directly against directives of his very own state governors and public health experts.

The situation became so grim that *The Brazilian Report*, an online news outlet, turned its hawkeyed gaze on the pandemic, releasing videos starkly showing just how bad the situation was. Bolsonaro wasn't exceptional to the virus, for he also suffered its wrath sometime in late July 2020 (Saraiva, 2020). Thousands of people contracted COVID-19, and thousands more weren't lucky enough to fight it off; instead, it took them with it to the mass graves.

The viral disease was so draining on every sector in all hospitals that everyone was devastatingly worn out and depressed. We heard of doctors, nurses, paramedics, and all other hospital workers dying, some taking their lives due to stress and mental torture, as in the case of Dr. Lorna Breen. By April, according to Al Jazeera, the world had been infected to the tune of over 3.1 million people in 185 countries. On the grim side, those who had fought for their lives and lost had reached over 224,600 people. On the bright side of things, there were 957,000 who had come out of the scourge, albeit weak but lucky to be alive (Al Jazeera, April 2020). One of those who lost their lives, according to *The Standard* daily newspaper, was a nurse in the United States who was unlucky to fight the virus out (*The Standard* Daily, 2020). In the United States alone, there were about 1 million infections by April 2020. The United States had reclaimed the global title of the COVID-19 pandemic hotbed of the world.

CHAPTER 12

Effects of COVID-19 on Education

A global phenomenon of COVID-19's kind had never been seen by modern generations, and it brought education to a halt the world over. Education at all levels starting from preschool to higher levels literally came to a standstill, mainly due to the fact that the pandemic was an unknown illness. Thus, institutions at all levels around the world closed doors and learning remained suspended for an unspecified period of time, with hopes that the virus would just disappear and never be felt again. Some leaders even verbalized this notion and remained adamant about the measure put in place by global health organizations.

However, what they failed to notice and see was that COVID-19 was a real phenomenon of a kind never seen or felt by modern generations, and it has proved to be here with us for the long haul. Based on the way these leaders behaved, even though they were old enough to borrow on experiences from history, it seemed they had never seen anything like it before. Case in point was the president of Brazil, who declared that COVID-19 was totally harmless! He refused to wear a face mask while in public gatherings. He called and attended many public meetings as though there was nothing happening in the world.

Some countries that attempted to reopen with strict measures in place immediately shut down due to the virus reemerging. This is because, when the virus takes root in an area, it spreads like bushfire. To avoid this, schools resorted to distant learning, online learning, and electronic learning (eLearning). Some opted for blended learning and others learning by correspondence.

In March 2020, school gates around the world slammed shut, leaving about 1.5 billion young people at home as part of a broader shutdown to protect people from the novel coronavirus. So far, because of these measures, there have been very few cases of COVID-19 in schools, especially among schoolchildren of lower elementary ages, between four and nine years old. One of the contributing factors may be that schools have remained closed as infections continue to ravage the general public. Also, it may likely be due to very little data relating to COVID-19 infections in children and not necessarily due to the fact that children may be less vulnerable or susceptible to the virus. The latter, therefore, may mean that the rate of infection in children is just as fast or just as high as that in adults, and that will remain a possibility until there is credible reliable data that shows otherwise. It may also mean that there is an aspect of this virus or a strength that children have that is advantageous to them—something that adults lack that keeps them strong.

Different theories have been floated about this strange but awesome phenomenon. The best science there is right now to help explain this is a study that was done looking at what are called the ACE2 receptors, which are how coronavirus gets into the body. The study, published in the *Journal of the American Medical Association (JAMA)*, looked at ACE2 gene expression in the nose; it was found that, in the youngest children, from ages four to nine years old, there was very little gene expression. To the contrary, there is more gene expression in the middle school and high school age group. Furthermore, there is the most gene expression in adults! This front-running study explains and reflects on the transmission patterns and how frequently children are getting it in those different age groups. This data and epidemiology, as well as basic viral science, clearly shows that high school-aged kids are the kids that you need to worry about going forward as schools and other public places plan to reopen for normal life.

So, we need to change our mentality going forward as relates to the notion that permeated into us that children are vectors or rather viral cesspools. Children don't get severe strains of the virus. Nor do they have a stronger immune system that shields them from the virus. However, it seems that, even in direct contact with infected people, children are unlikely to be infected as easily as earlier thought. Carriers are very dangerous to their families, especially to the elderly—such as grandmothers and grandfathers living with their families—so children could have infected their parents, if they were carriers.

Apart from this, there are other vulnerabilities that affect children's education and actually may completely alter the progress, as well as the quantity and quality of education, not to mention access to it. Some of these issues that have reared their ugly heads influenced by the outbreak of the CIVID-19 pandemic include all manner of abuses of children, such as teenage pregnancies, physical child abuse, forced child marriages, female genital mutilation and sexual abuses of both boys and girls, hunger, and lack of psychosocial support available at school in terms of children's interactions with others and guidance from teachers. These cases have exposed underlying simmering problems that have dogged families for a long time but have been exacerbated by COVID-19. These issues are definitely going to widen the gap of inequalities between the rich and the poorest of societies.

These issues add to the wounds of girls and boys living with disabilities, literally! Unfortunately, they live in some of the poorest families and face discrimination in their communities. They generally are not prioritized in terms of their right to an education. During this COVID-19 pandemic, things won't be better for them either; they are going to face an even higher risk of exclusion in all spheres of life, the education sphere being no exception.

The consequences of these issues are compounding day by day and are dire to the society at large, especially to the African society, where there are no strict laws to combat these vices. We cannot turn a blind eye either to the fact that these consequences are long term and are going to hurt society at large and cause retrogression for decades to come. Governments should robustly pursue perpetrators of the aforementioned atrocities to children and bring them to book. This will send a strong message to parents to be vigilant, as well as to the molesters to shun their evil ways.

So what options are educators left with to carry on with their noble profession? The most affected sector as far as we know due to the COVID-19 pandemic, educators are struggling to take different approaches to further their work. In an effort to mitigate the short- and long-term impact of school closures on learners and ensure continued learning, many governments globally have adopted some form of distance learning. However, the results of these efforts are far from ideal, as the many challenges, especially in developing countries, are countless. These challenges assocoated with romote education eventually denies educational accessibility to majority of the learners.

Children living in remote areas are the most affected, though the trend is general. Some limiting factors include access to internet connection (or lack thereof). For those in rural areas, the challenge is multifold; there may be no infrastructure close to the needy. If such infrastructure does exist, the expense may be financially crushing, rendering children unable to afford to access the internet. For others, even though they may be able to access the internet, they can only do so if they have the electronics needed, which are usually pricey as well—not to mention the expense that normally comes with maintenance of gadgets and powering them, which may be prohibitive as well. On top of that, these electronic gadgets may not survive in harsh dry and sandy environments, even for those who do have the expertise to maintain them.

Plus, there are also the issues of managing the learners and the learning process so that learners can hunker down and get to learning. The results are far from ideal, as distance learning courses are not accessible to the majority of leaners. So, before we'll be able to provide the really vulnerable learners in remote areas with internet, laptops, tablets or smartphones, and TVs or radios, governments will have to build the infrastructure, train teachers how to use it, provide funding for continued maintenance, and provide continued moral and financial support to teachers and learners alike.

CHAPTER 13

Traditional Exorcism of COVID-19 Evil Spirits in Kenya

Disease, especially a disease that has no cure or remedy or that is emerging anew, arouses in people a lot of mixed feelings and a turmoil of emotions, among them fear, anxiety, stress, depression, and rage. And this causes many unreasonable, unintentional, outrageous, uncalled for, shocking, and nerve-racking reactions from all and sundry. Therefore, the very strange happenings we hear about—a mother poisoning her four children, another mother tying up all her children and tossing them into a deep river and finally tossing herself in, all four drowning; a husband and wife deciding to drink disinfectant to their death; a president of a particular country endorsing an herbal concoction as a treatment for COVID-19; or traditional African elders being held up in a forest exorcising evil COVID-19 spirits so the disease will mysteriously disappear—are very shocking but, at the same time, understandable to a certain degree.

We all of us are very different from each other and respond differently. It is usually said that we all are madmen and madwomen and that only the degree of madness differs.

Therefore, we need to be dealing with each other with care and kindness! The effects of a disease can expose or exacerbate an individual's mental condition, even when someone has never shown signs of a mental condition before. This could have been the case with a woman called Mwende from Kenya, who killed her four children by poisoning them all at the same time. On the same fateful day, the woman went looking for her ex-boyfriend at a nearby town, Naivasha, failing to find him. Before she left, she told the court that she left him a letter that she'd written in a daze. She was said to have had no food to feed her children due to the effects of COVID-19. The church leaders who attended the funeral of the four children admitted that COVID-19 had taken a tall on the population, voicing the need for people to bear the happenings with fortitude. According to one by the name of Mr. Mwaura, families were going through hard times, but those affected should not suffer in silence. He said that the pandemic had affected the social setup and people's incomes but encouraged any with problems to reach out to friends and family and to pour their hearts out for help.

In another separate sad COVID-19-related case in Arizona, in the United States, a husband and wife poisoned themselves trying to self-medicate with chloroquine phosphate. The chemical is used to treat parasite in fish. According to NBC News, the couple, both in their sixties, had listened to President Donald Trump's insistence that chloroquine, a decade-old antimalaria drug as a very promising treatment for COVID-19 (Hillyard and Edwards, 2020). The couple misunderstood the president and mixed a small amount of the chloroquine phosphate with a certain liquid before drinking the solution. In just twenty minutes both became ill. The woman started vomiting, and the man developed a severe respiratory problem. They called 9-1-1, and soon after arriving at the hospital, the man died of cardiac arrest. The woman was initially in critical condition but became stable and fully recovered afterward.

Because of fear, anxiety, and stress about what might happen if we get infected by the disease, people rush to actions with the intentions of saving themselves. These actions, whatever they may be, could prove to be fatal, either to the person him or herself or to close family members. It is important to seek a second opinion where possible, for example in the chloroquine case, rather than going ahead with such a plan.

A strange Indian "holy" man from Ratlam in Madhya Pradesh claimed that he could perform an exorcism to cure his followers and others who had COVID-19. He actually failed to protect himself from the virus's ruthless ravaging effects, got infected, and died of the virus sometime in early June. According to *The Sauce*, the exorcist would kiss the hands of devotees and tell them that the kissing would keep them free from the virus (The Sauce: Lifestyle, 2020). To the contrary, contact tracing has revealed that he ended up infecting twenty of his followers. Despite the virus spreading through contagious droplets from the mouth and nose, he strangely called his kissing the "kiss cure." Health officials confirmed that the man tested positive on June 3, 2020, and had died twenty-four hours later.

In another strange exorcist case in the West African country of the Ivory Coast, an Ivorian traditional group performed a special exorcism ceremony, seeking divine intervention to protect its population of three million people from the coronavirus epidemic. In an odd statement from the king, it was claimed that the monarch could order a procession of naked women to ward off coronavirus by seeking the protection of spirits. According to Africanews, the chief of Swani, King Amon N'Douffou V, said, "I ask God … to protect the population and keep this virus away from the kingdom, Ivory Coast and the

World." The king spoke through his official announcer, as the royals do not address the public directly. While speaking at the ceremony, he alluded to divine instructions underlying the pandemic "because science can't fix everything. It just can't. Take for example the virus, this little virus that we don't see that silences everybody (AfricaNews, 2020)."

He went on to say, "Those that we call powerful, less powerful and so on, everybody is at the same level. Today if everybody hides, we are weak. This is a message that God is giving to us," he stressed (Africanews, 2020).

Traditional kings and local chieftains have great authority, and the event would normally have been attended by hundreds of people. However, due to coronavirus restrictions, Africanews reveals that the ceremony was held within restrictions, keeping the gathering to less than fifty participants and showing that the group had imposed containment measures, as is the case across much of Africa.

The traditional *kimians*, or women healers, dressed in white purified the royal court by sprinkling alcohol to the strains of the *abodan*, a traditional beat. Those attending then daubed their faces with the wet earth as a sign of obeisance to the chief and lifted their heads toward the sun. According to Africanews, such ceremonies are held from time to time to ward off natural disasters, such as drought, floods, or diseases.

Records indicates that about 20 percent of the population of Ivory Coast is animist. Muslims and Christians account for 40 percent of the religious population each, and many members of the two faiths also practice traditional beliefs alongside their faiths.

CHAPTER 14

Men versus Women: Who Is the COVID-19 Weaker Sex?

A surprising medical observation was deduced from the data collected over the few months of COVID-19 pandemic havoc. It showed that men had been under siege of the virus and were highly susceptible to it. According to a study published in the *Annals of Internal Medicine*, men surpassed women by about half in numbers of those infected by coronavirus previously (Joffe H. et al., 2020). It looks like the differences in infection observed in the sexes are founded in the underlying basic strength inherent in the sexes. Over the years, studies have shown that girls have a lower infant mortality than boys, meaning that the chances of baby girl's surviving after birth are higher. No wonder this phenomenon is not so surprising but rather replicated throughout life! It is even known in the general global population. It is not definitively known why women are stronger than men health-wise, but a number of theories have been postulated.

According to the US National Library of Medicine; National Institutes of Health, at the cellular level, a major difference is that female cells have two X chromosomes, whereas male cells have a single X and a single Y chromosome (Maleki Dana et al., 2020). It has been proven that the answer is in the X chromosome, which plays a major role in boosting women's immune system. Given that men have a single X chromosome and women two, it is logical why women exhibit stronger immune systems than men attributed to these differences. This is partly the reason the population of women has historically been higher than that of men globally. Naturally, women are a stronger species than men in terms of the body fighting diseases. Although the influence of cellular differences between males and females on the infectious disease process is not fully understood, it is known that the X chromosome governs many of the immune system responses in the human body, unlike the Y chromosome.

It is also believed that behavioral factors have a lot to do with these trends. Women are viewed to be more cautious with their cleanliness than men; thus, women wash their hands more often than do men. Around the house, women tend to be better at keeping their floors, countertops, tabletops, chairs, utensils, and other things around the house clean than are men. Bearing in mind the fact that coronavirus exists on different objects for a while before it dies, it follows, therefore, that men may contract it from contaminated objects more often than women do. Studies have also shown that men are less likely to wash their hands or that, when they do, they are less likely to use soap, unlike women. On the other side, in the process of cleaning, women keep their hands clean longer than do men. At the same time, when they are pushed to, men wait longer before washing their hands and, even worse, see it as a weakness for them.

Lastly but not least, men are foolhardy! When they are infected by any kind of disease, they tend to take longer to see a doctor than do women, unless they are pushed by their partners, friends, or family. Women, on the other hand, are the direct opposite in terms of that tendency. They are quick to talk about health issues to their family and friends and also seek medical intervention quickly and on their own.

However, men are not to be blamed. Their behavior is due to the societal expectations or norms that insist on portraying men as the "stronger sex" over women; hence, seeking medical treatment or assistance is viewed as a sign of weakness.

CHAPTER 15

Travel Restrictions, Lockdowns, and Other Measures

Global travel was the first to be hard hit, especially travel from Asian countries to the rest of the world. One incredible thing that amazed me was airline travel. As countries continued to impose lockdowns, so did flights; tight restrictions were put in place. This came with varying levels of clearances from governments around the world. Case in point, on February 28, 2020, a Chinese airplane with 239 passengers landed at Jomo Kenyatta International Airport in Kenya amid a huge uproar from Kenyans. The plane sneaked into the country but was uncovered by one of the concerned workers on duty that day. This was a time when the effects and even the full symptoms of COVID-19 were not known. Kenyans, having been enlightened about the dangers of the virus, flooded social media to express their displeasure over the reopening of its air space.

Alongside the travel restrictions came the inevitable economic shrinkage and downturn. We generally know that infrastructural development is the engine of economic development. Also, a lot of investments have been put into this infrastructure. So even having them lying idle is a waste of resources. It is therefore really hard to wrap the mind around the thought of all airplanes lying around hangars and other makeshift storage units around the world. Flying spurs all other forms of movement—may it be vehicular transportation or movement on trains, bicycles, or motorbikes to get people to their final destinations so that they can get on with national building activities.

To reduce and curb the economic hemorrhage due to the pandemic, governments around the world injected money into their economies in various trenches in the form of stimulus packages. For instance, in the United States, Congress passed several major pieces of legislation responding to the COVID-19 pandemic in the month of March. The government released a total of about $3 trillion as the CARES Act in phases, starting with $8.3 billion for phase one—health agencies and initial small business loans. Phase two released COVID-19 relief amounting to $100 billion was passed on March 17, 2020, which was mainly for paid sick leave, unemployment benefits, and food assistance. Then there was phase three, which was the biggest of them all and was passed on the same day as phase two. It was meant for the Coronavirus Aid, Relief, and Economic Security (CARES) Act. This amounted to $2 trillion in tax credit, making the stimulus packages an equivalent of 45 percent of all 2019 federal spending. According to USAFacts, the first tier of COVID-19 release support went to families to the tune of $1,200 for every family based on their income to a certain level (USAFacts, 2020). For each dependent in a family, an additional $600 was given to that family. The identification of the families was based on the 2019 tax return.

In Kenya, the United Nation's World Food Program (WFP), in conjunction with the government of Kenya, launched cash transfers and nutritional food support for more than a quarter million people struggling to survive from the impact of COVID-19 in informal settlements in the capital city of Nairobi. The assistance came from other UN partners, including the United States, Finland, Poland, and Sweden; WFP continues to assist 279,000 people in Nairobi's informal settlement with cash transfers and nutritional support. Each family from informal settlements such as Kibra, Mukuru, Kariobangi, Mathare, and a few others without any income received US$ 40 every month for three months to help cover their daily basic needs.

To aim for the youth, the government introduced a program to help them. Under this program, unlike the informal settlement initiative, in which families got money without conditions, the Kazi Kwa Vijana Mtaani Initiative Program enabled youths to be occupied by cleaning and beautifying their neighborhoods. In turn, they could at least earn US$ 550 every month for their work. This program was intended to cushion and keep youth (defined as the most vulnerable yet able-bodied citizens in the informal settlements) busy to prevent them from getting into drug peddling or, even worse, drug use. The first phase of Kazi Kwa Vijana Initiative focused in Nairobi, Mombasa, Kiambu, Nakuru, Kisumu, Kilifi, Kwale, and Mandera.

CHAPTER 16

The Natural Remedies That Many Take for Granted

These remedies that have been shared world over might look simple and cheap. But believe me, they are the sure remedies, or medication if you will. They are 100 percent approved by every medical expert around the world. Used before infection these remedies reduce the impact of COVID-19 to the body. On the other hand, used after the infection, these remedies quicken recovery by boosting the immune system providing immence comfort to the body. This is important since COVID-19 patients feel belaboured due to the deprivation of oxyen in the body. The remedies help in the absorbtion of the oxygen.

When sick, many look for sophisticated medical solutions in a desperate effort to get well quick. In the initial stages, this virus is so intrussive to the body yet so evasive, then it's really agressive in intensity once it's taken hold of the body. Also, as mentioned above, the virus leaves the infected with devastating side effects / injury that may not be immediately felt but might last for a very long time before disappearing, if not remaining permanently. It is said, prevention is better than cure! So, why not just prevent the virus from taking hold, rather than suffer the pain of trauma, rejection, and profiling, not to mention death?

Now, without further ado, the first remedy is *so* easy— so much that it is made up of easily available food items commonly found in our houses and markets. One just needs lemons, garlic, ginger, and clean water to fix a nice, easy-to-take concoction that surely will keep the virus spread in the body in check. Boil this for thirty to forty-five minutes, let it cool for some time, and then take it warm or hot. The other amazing thing about this archaic medicinal remedy is that there is no limit or dosage to worry about, unlike with other modern conventional remedies we know of.

Many people either do not know about this remedy, or outrightly ignore it as useless or inconsequential. The remedy is not that pricey; neither are the items it's made from, especially in comparison to the high-end, specialized medical attention we've been accustomed to seeing or hearing about COVID-19 patients getting since the virus hit us. With this, there is no being bedridden, no ventilators and no oxygenation needed, no pain pills involved, and no dosage of some sort or another. Simply visit your local market or mama mboga (street grocery woman), get the items, and come home and fix them.

So simple yet so powerful, this remedy has actually saved many from being bedridden, including famous iconic anchor Jeff Koinange, who actually contracted the virus, had to quarantine at home for two weeks, and went back to work stronger than ever. Every time you saw Jeff on Citizen TV working from home, he had a mug of the concoction, which he sipped from time to time. In a Youtube video interviewed by Victoria Rubadiri of Kenya Citizen TV Jeff narated how effective the concoction in keeping him hydrated apart ftom nuirishing him (Rubadiri, 2020).

Another confirmation comes from Foreign Affairs Permanent Secretary Macharia Kamau, who also contacted the virus. Kamau said that he took the concoction several times a day, and it actually helped him boost his immune system.

However, Dr. Patrick Amoth, who is the acting director at the Ministry of Health in Kenya, while speaking during one of the COVID-19 press briefings, insisted that the concoction—which is ginger, lemon, honey, and garlic—is not an instant cure for the disease. Amoth said, "Ginger, lemon and honey are good because they are sources of vitamins and micronutrients, but the message to take home today is that there is still no cure for COVID-19. I will not stop you from taking your ginger, honey and lemon as many times as you want but for sure it is not a treatment for COVID-19." Dr. Omoth's message was specifically geared toward enforcing the preventive measures put in place by the Kenyan Government and not necessarily disaproving the power of the remedies.

People have used this remedy since time immemorial, with various additional variations of fruits and vegetables in addition to the four essential items. When making this delicious concoction, always use fresh ginger, fresh lemon, fresh garlic, and raw natural honey, rather than artificial or powdered products from a bottle. Take your ginger and cut it to a piece that you think will be enough for you. Take a mortar and a pestle and grind the ginger until it becomes fine. After that, remove it with a spoon and set it aside. Peel four cloves of garlic as well and grind it in the mortar. Then set it aside by the ginger. Put a cooking pot with water on the heat. Add the garlic and the ginger to the water in the cooking pot. Allow it to simmer for ten minutes before you remove it. Once it's ready, pour it in a cup, and then cut your lemon in half and squeeze the lemon juice into the mixture in the cup. It's at this point that you can add a tablespoon of raw honey. If you like it, you can add in a pinch of cinnamon for flavor. At this point you're ready to consume the concoction. Remember to take it while it's still warm, or hot if you prefer.

Alternatively, if you like a bitter flavor, mix the chopped ginger, garlic, and lemon with peels into a cooking pot and leave it to simmer. Fill your cup and add honey to taste and drink hot or warm.

Well, the concoction is not one of those commercials that promises to be "the cure that doctors don't want you to know"; it's not that kind of thing! This is a universally open secret, and the items involved are used daily in our lives. We can use these items for our benefit this time to slowly try to bring the COVID-19 global pandemic to a halt. What could probably hold us back is the price of the items, which is going up as many people discover the effectiveness of the remedy.

It is important to note and even warn readers that as much as these remedies effectively work, testing and seeking professional medical diagnosis is not a choice but part and percel of the treatment process to ensure that you are actually infected and treating COVID-19 and not some other ailment. Also, the earlier you test, discover the disease and start the remedy the better and the more effective it works! It is therefore encouraged that testing as soon as you feel unwell and getting professional medical advice be of priority, before starting the remedy. However, there is no dossage that goes with this remedy and therefor taking the concoction however much can never be harmful. NOTE: Never take or use the remedy if you have an allergy to any of the items used to prepare the concoction.

Another fantastic way to get rid of this Coronavirus is by a steaming therapy or rather the COVID TONIC. Steam therapy was used on me by my mother long before I knew what it was. Nevertheless, it is highly advisable to seek medical diagnoses if you feel sick or suspect you have been in contact with a COVID-19 victim before you use this remedy. What you need for this remedy is about 3 liters of water, a whole onion, 4 cloves of garlic, about 250 grams ginger or fist full-scraped or thoroughly washed, and 1 large lemon. Chop them all and put them in the water in a pot and boil them for about an hour. Take the pot from the stove as it steams and place it on a stable stand or floor. Get a towel and cover your head completely over the hot COVID TONIC pot. You will inhale the steam till the water cools down. You can take short breaks if you feel uncomfortable to relax. Lemon is very rich in Vitamin C; however, it becomes alkaline when boiled. The COVID-19 virus does not survive/like alkaline environment, so it is killed. Ginger is very rich in Zinc which helps to boost your immune system. Garlic contains a lot of medicinal benefits. Infact, back in the days ginger was used for anesthetic and antibacterial purposes. Onions have a lot of antibacterial properties that help fight bacteria. When boiled in water, all those properties are released and carried into the steam and when inhaled they pass through your nostril, mouth, down your throat and breathing system and into the lungs. This process is recommended three times a day. Also, before steaming yourself, put some in a cup aside for drinking. Drink at least two cups a day of the COVID tonic warm or hot. One cup in the morning and another in the evening. COVID-19 does not survive well in hot or warm environments and that combination of high temperature and the COVID TONIC helps clear it out. Over time doing this boosts the immune system and helps speed the recovery process. As stressed, before you embark on this remedy you must have been diagnosed or seen by a doctor for COVID-19 medical diagnoses. The steam therapy has been used to fight bacterial, common cold and other viruses for a very long time. It is completely 100% natural, it is cheap or almost cheap and it's tried and tested for 3500 years according to FGB Natural

Products (Fastdesign, 2020). Respiratory benefits of steam therapy include:

- Moisturiser dry, irritated nasal and throat passages making them more comfortable
- Alleviates soreness and inflammation of the throat
- Liquefies mucus secretions, resulting in clearer secretions that are easier to expel by coughing or blowing the nose
- Relaxes throat muscles, reducing the cough reflex
- Dilates blood vessels, encouraging better blood flow and overall circulation

There are four ways that one can administer Steam Therapy. The traditional way explained above, through inhalation equipment, by shower or by steaming equipment. Above is one my parents restrained me in even before I knew its medicinal importance. I am thankful to them, it made me the strong healthy man I am. I was forcefully held in that steamer until all the hard smelly dirt on my body stripped off with the sweat from the steamer.

BIBLIOGRAPHY

Africanews. "Ivorian Group Holds Exorcism Ceremony against Virus." March 5, 2020. Accessed December 11, 2020. https://www.africanews.com/2020/05/03/ivorian-group-holds-exorcism-ceremony-against-virus//.

BBC News. "Coronavirus: Outcry after Trump Suggests Injecting Disinfectant as Treatment." April 24, 2020. Accessed December 13, 2020. https://www.bbc.com/news/world-us-canada-52407177.

Centers for Disease Control and Prevention. "Vaccine Effectiveness: How Well Do The Flu Vaccines Work?" January 3, 2020. Accessed December 12, 2020. https://www.cdc.gov/flu/vaccines-work/vaccineeffect.htm.

Christensen, Jen. "Three Simple Acts Can Stop COVID-19 Outbreaks, Study Finds." *CNN*, July 22, 2020. Accessed December 8, 2020. https://www.cnn.com/2020/07/21/health/covid-19-three-things-will-stop-it-wellness/index.html.

COVID-19: Rise in the Number of Cases and Deaths. Accessed December 8, 2020. https://interactive.afp.com/graphics/COVID-19-Rise-in-the-number-of-cases-and-deaths_600/.

Crist, Carolyn. "Study Uncovers Six COVID-19 Symptom Clusters." *WebMD*, July 29. 2020. Accessed December 8, 2020. https://www.webmd.com/lung/

news/20200729/study-uncovers-six-coicd-19-symptom-clusters#:~:text=Here%20are%20the%20six%20clusters,hoarseness%2C%20fever%2C%20loss%20of%20appetite.

Dartnell, Lewis. "The Covid-19 changes that could last long-term." *BBC Future*, June 29, 2020. Accessed 9 December, 2020. https://www.bbc.com/future/article/20200629-which-lockdown-changes-are-here-to-stay.

Edwards, Erika, and Vaughn Hillyard. "Man Dies after Taking Chloroquine in an Attempt to Prevent Coronavirus." *NBC News*, March 23, 2020. Accessed December 9, 2020. https://www.nbcnews.com/health/health-news/man-dies-after-ingesting-chloroquine-attempt-prevent-coronavirus-n1167166.

FGB. "Three Powerful Reasons to Use Steam Therapy for Colds." May 29, 2020. Accessed December 9, 2020. https://www.fgb.com.au/blog/cold-and-flu/3-powerful-reasons-use-steam-therapy-colds.

Gates, Bill. "What You Need to Know about the COVID-19 Vaccine." *GatesNotes*, April 30, 2020. Accessed December 8, 2020. https://www.gatesnotes.com/Health/What-you-need-to-know-about-the-COVID-19-vaccine.

Gavi. "Do Lockdowns Actually Work?" June 12, 2020. Accessed June 28, 2020. https://www.gavi.org/vaccineswork/do-lockdowns-actually-work.

King's College London. "Six Distinct 'Types' of COVID-19 Identified." July 17, 2020. Accessed December 9, 2020. https://www.kcl.ac.uk/news/six-distinct-types-of-covid-19-identified.

Koinange, Jeff. "This Thing Is Real! Jeff Koinange Gives His Story in Self-Isolation." Video. *Kenya Citizen TV*, July 22, 2020. https://www.youtube.com/watch?v=Y2yx8tp91KA.

Maleki Dana, Parisa, Fatemeh Sadoughi, Jamal Hallajzadeh, Zatollah Asemi, Mohammad Ali Mansournia, Bahman

Yousefi, and Mansooreh Momen-Heravi. 2020. "An Insight into the Sex Differences in COVID-19 Patients: What are the Possible Causes?" *Preshop Disaster Med.* Accessed December 11, 2020. https://www.ncbi.nlm.nih.gov/pmc/articles/PMC7327162/#:~:text=Sex%20Differences%20in%20Inflammatory%20Processes&text=Plasma%20concentration%20of%20testosterone%2C%20which,obesity%2C%20and%20obstructive%20sleep%20apnea.&text=Evidence%20has%20shown%20that%2.

McKay, Betsy, and Daniela Hernandez. "Coronavirus Hijacks the Body From Head to Toe, Perplexing Doctors." *The Wall Street Journal*, May 7, 2020. Accessed December 9, 2020. https://www.wsj.com/articles/coronavirus-hijacks-the-body-from-head-to-toe-perplexing-doctors-11588864248.

McNamara, Audrey. "Multiple Vaccine Doses Could Be Necessary to Protect from Coronavirus, Bill Gates Says." *CBS News*, July 23, 2020. Accessed December 8, 2020. https://www.cbsnews.com/news/coronavirus-vaccine-bill-gates-multiple-doses/.

Melinek, Judy. "When Did COVID-19 Arrive and Could We Have Spotted It Earlier?" *MedPage Today*, May 4, 2020. Accessed December 8, 2020. https://www.medpagetoday.com/blogs/working-stiff/86291.

Nation. "Steroid Breakthrough Raises Virus Hopes, Despite China Outbreak." June 16, 2020. Accessed December 10, 2020. https://nation.africa/kenya/news/world/steroid-breakthrough-raises-virus-hopes-despite-china-outbreak-685798.

Page, Jeremy, Wenxin Fan, and Natasha Khan. "How It All Started: China's Early Coronavirus Missteps." *The Wall Street Journal*, March 6, 2020. Accessed December 10,

2020. https://www.wsj.com/articles/how-it-all-starte
d-chinas-early-coronavirus-missteps-11583508932.

Saraiva, Augusta. "Field Hospitals Are Preventing a Healthcare
Collapse in Brazil." *The Brazilian Report*, May 4, 2020.
Accessed December 11, 2020. https://brazilian.report/
society/2020/05/04/field-hospitals-are-preventing-
a-healthcare-collapse-in-brazil/.

Spagnolo, Primavera A., JoAnn E. Manson, and Hadine Joffe.
2020. "Sex and Gender Differences in Health: What the
COVID-19 Pandemic Can Teach Us." *Annals of Internal
Medicine.* Accessed December 11, 2020. https://www.
acpjournals.org/doi/10.7326/M20-1941.

Tanui, Nikko. "No Reunion Yet for Brenda, Family Say They
Are Still Cautious." *The Standard*, April 3, 2020. Accessed
December 8, 2020. https://www.standardmedia.co.ke/
nairobi/article/2001366702/why-brenda-will-not-mee
t-family-soon-despite-recovering-from-virus.

The Jerusalem Post. "COVID-19 Is Weakening, Could Die
Out without Vaccine, Specialist Claims." June 22, 2020.
Accessed December 9, 2020. https://www.jpost.com/
health-science/covid-19-is-weakening-could-die-out-w
ithout-vaccine-specialist-claims-632324.

The Sauce. "Weird World: Indian Exorcist Dies Of COVID-19."
June 15, 2020. Accessed December 11, 2020. https://
www.capitalfm.co.ke/thesauce/weird-world-india
n-exorcist-dies-of-covid-19/.

"Two Makeshift Hospitals just Opened in New York City to
Help Battle the Coronavirus Pandemic." Video. *CNBC*,
April 1, 2020. https://www.cnbc.com/video/2020/04/01/
coronavirus-two-makeshift-hospitals-just-opened-
in-new-york-city.html.

USA Facts. "The $2 Trillion CARES Act, a Response
to COVID-19, Is Equivalent to 45 Percent of All
2019 Federal Spending." April 5, 2020. Accessed

December 11, 2020. https://usafacts.org/articles/
what-will-cares-act-and-other-congressional-corona
virus-bills-do-how-big-are-they/#:~:text=On%20
March%2027%2C%202020%2C%20the,federal%20
government%20expenditures%20in%202019.

WHO Coronavirous Disease (COVID-19) Dashboard. Accessed
December 10, 2020. https://covid19.who.int/.

Williams, Terri-Ann. "There Are Six 'Types' of Covid-19 – and
Each Cause a Different 'Cluster of Symptoms,' Scientists
Reveal." *The U.S. Sun*, July 17, 2020. Accessed December 8,
2020. https://www.the-sun.com/news/1156699/six-type
s-covid-19-each-causes-different-cluster-symptoms/.

Zhang, Sarah. "A Vaccine Reality Check." *The Atlantic*,
July 24, 2020. Accessed December 10, 2020. https://
www.theatlantic.com/health/archive/2020/07/
covid-19-vaccine-reality-check/614566/.

ABOUT THE AUTHOR

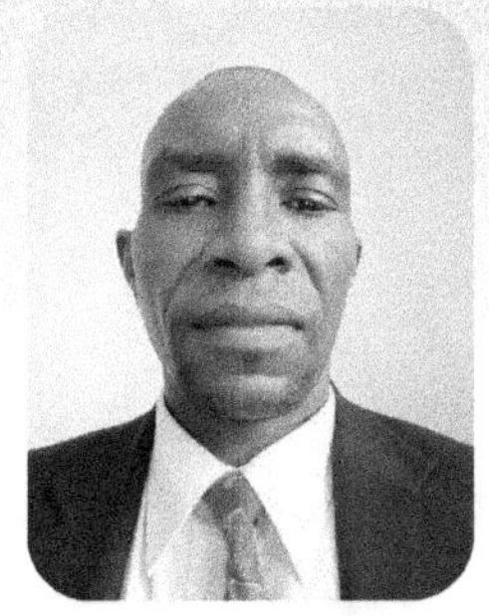

Evans Lugalia Mudanya was born in western Kenya. He trained as a teacher at Kaimosi Teacher Training College in Kenya and taught in various Kenya elementary schools for five years. In 2001, he moved to the United States and studied at Kirkwood Community College graduating with an AA Degree in 2004. He continued to University of Northern Iowa (UNI) Business School graduating with BA in Management of information Systems (MIS). He then joined Graduate school for an MA in Instructional Technology from UNI College of Education. He joined Lincoln University Graduate School in Oakland California, where he enrolled for a DBA in Finance and Investments but did not finish. Mudanya and his two children; a boy and a girl live in the US.